KETOGEN

Ketogenic Diet Recipes That You Can Prepare Using 7 Ingredients and Less in Less Than 30 Minutes

(With Pictures)

Your Free Gifts

As a way of thanking you for the purchase, I'd like to offer you 2 complimentary gifts:

- **How To Get Through Any Weight Loss Plateau While On The Ketogenic Diet:** The title is self-explanatory; if you are struggling with getting off a weight loss plateau while on the Keto diet, you will find this free gift very eye opening on what has been ailing you. Grab your copy now by clicking/tapping here or simply enter http://bit.ly/2fantonpubketo into your browser.

- **5 Pillar Life Transformation Checklist:** This short book is about life transformation, presented in bit size pieces for easy implementation. I believe that without such a checklist, you are likely to have a hard time implementing anything in this book and any other thing you set out to do religiously and sticking to it for the long haul. It doesn't matter whether your goals relate to weight loss, relationships, personal finance, investing, personal development, improving communication in your family, your overall health, finances, improving your sex life, resolving issues in your relationship, fighting PMS successfully, investing, running a successful business, traveling etc. With a checklist like this one, you can bet that anything you do will seem a lot easier to implement until the end. Therefore, even if you don't continue reading this book, at least read the one thing that will help you in every other aspect of your life. Grab your copy now by clicking/tapping here or simply enter http://bit.ly/2fantonfreebie into your browser. Your life will never be the same again (if you implement what's in this book), I promise.

PS: I'd like your feedback. If you are happy with this book, please leave a review on Amazon.

Introduction

The Ketogenic diet is the King of all diets and for a good reason; no other diet delivers benefits like the keto diet without putting dieters in the awkward position of fighting off hunger. While it actually over-delivers, many people have a hard time following it because of information overload.

By this, I mean, while there are tons of recipes to prepare to follow the Ketogenic diet easily, not many of us have the passion and commitment to prepare recipes that require over 10 different ingredients several times a week. It can get way too costly for many average dieters. Worse still, some recipes require too much time to prepare. It is not uncommon to find recipes that take as much as 1 hour, 2 hours or more. How are you supposed to prepare these in a working week? All this can be a real deal breaker for many dieters, as many of us these days hardly have time left from our busy schedules, which explains why buying take-outs seems like the easiest and most practical thing to do.

That's why I wrote this book after seeing the problems that many dieters experienced after being on the Ketogenic diet. After my wife had a problem finding recipes that she could prepare without wanting to pull off her hair because they are complicated and take too much time, I realized that I needed to find something for her to follow. And that's when I ventured into finding recipes that other dieters can prepare in as little as 30 minutes.

So if you are looking for a quick summary to the Ketogenic diet along with tons of recipes that you can prepare with as little as 7 ingredients and in less than 30 minutes, this book is for you!

In this book, you will find:

1: A comprehensive description of the Ketogenic diet including

- ✓ *What it is*
- ✓ ***How it works***
- ✓ *Why it works*
- ✓ ***The benefits that come with following the keto diet***
- ✓ *What to eat while on the Ketogenic diet*
- ✓ ***What not to eat while on the Ketogenic diet***
- ✓ *How to get into ketosis*
- ✓ *And much more*

2: Over 70 Ketogenic diet recipes to help you get started including:

- ✓ *Breakfast recipes you can prepare with 7 ingredients or less in 30 minutes or less*
- ✓ ***Lunch recipes you can prepare with 7 ingredients or less in 30 minutes or less***

- ✓ *Dinner recipes you can prepare with 7 ingredients or less in 30 minutes or less*

- ✓ ***Dessert recipes you can prepare with 7 ingredients or less in 30 minutes or less***

- ✓ *Snack recipes you can prepare with 7 ingredients or less in 30 minutes or less*

3: And much, much more!

Let's get started.

Copyright 2018 by Fantonpublishers.com - All rights reserved.

Table of Contents

Your Free Gifts --- 2

Introduction --- 4

A Comprehensive Overview of the Ketogenic Diet- 15

What is Keto Diet? -- 15

Benefits of Ketogenic Diet -------------------------------- 21
- *1. Facilitate weight loss* ---------------------------- 21
- *2. Help Monitor Blood Sugar* --------------------- 22

What To Eat On Keto ----------------------------------- 26
- *1. Fats and Oils* ----------------------------------- 26
- *2. Veggies* -- 27
- *3. Proteins* --- 29
- *4. Nuts & Seeds* ---------------------------------- 30
- *5. Fruits* -- 31
- *6. Beverages* -------------------------------------- 32
- *7. Dairy products* -------------------------------- 33
- *8. Condiments and sweeteners* ----------------- 34

Foods to Avoid --- 35
- *1. Sugary foods* ---------------------------------- 35
- *2. Sugary beverages* ---------------------------- 36
- *3. Grains and corn* ------------------------------ 37

    4. Starchy tubers and veggies ------------------- *39*

    5. Legumes -- *40*

Keto Recipes with 7 Ingredients or Less That You Can Prepare Within 30 Minutes ------------------- 42

Breakfast Recipes ----------------------------------- 42

5-Ingredient Keto Mug Lasagna-------------------- 42

    Flaxseed Muffin in a Mug ------------------------ *44*

    Sugar-Free Lemon Mug Cake -------------------- *46*

    Vanilla Keto Mug Cake --------------------------- *48*

    One-Minute Keto Mug Bread -------------------- *50*

    Ketogenic Cloud Eggs----------------------------- *52*

    Bell Pepper Eggs ---------------------------------- *54*

    Bacon Egg Muffin Cups -------------------------- *56*

    Keto Mushroom Omelet -------------------------- *58*

    Frittata with Tomatoes and Cheese -------------- *60*

    Fast Fat Herbed Omelet -------------------------- *62*

    Bacon and Brie Frittata -------------------------- *64*

Lunches -- 66

    Orange and Sage Glazed Duck Breast ---------- *66*

    10-Minute Instant Pot Salmon------------------- *68*

    Ahi Tuna Poke Recipe---------------------------- *70*

    Shake and Bake Pork Chop ---------------------- *72*

    Chili Roasted Chicken Thighs -------------------- *74*

- Garlic Ghee Pan-Fried Cod — 75
- Prosciutto Melon Wrap-Ups — 77
- Basil Spinach Salad — 78
- Beef, Scallions and Red Bell Pepper Sauté — 79
- Fresh Tuna Salad — 80
- Goat Cheese & Spinach Salad — 81
- 5-Minute Keto Sardines Salad — 83

Dinner — 84
- Rosemary Garlic Chicken Kabobs — 84
- Low Carb Pork Medallions — 86
- Pesto Chicken with Mozzarella Casserole — 87
- Spinach and Bacon Salad — 89
- Instant Pot Steamed Crab Legs — 90
- Garlic Butter Brazilian Steak — 91
- Jalapeno Cheddar Burgers — 93
- Easy Buffalo Wings — 95
- Baked Bacon Cheddar Meatballs — 97
- Low carb Skillet Lasagna — 99
- Low-Carb Pesto Baked Sea Bass — 101
- Bunless Low Carb Burger — 103

Snacks — 105
- Cucumber Spinach Smoothie — 105
- Avocado Salsa — 107

Black Beauty – Low Carb Vodka Drink --------109
Keto Dairy Free Shamrock ---------------------- 111
Asparagus and Leek Soup ----------------------- 112
Low Carb Strawberry Margarita Gummy Worms -- 114
Salmon and Cream Cheese Bites ---------------- 116
Vanilla Pumpkin Seed Clusters ----------------- 118
Pan-Fried Asparagus -----------------------------120
Low Carb Egg Salad ------------------------------ 121
Ketogenic Egg Cups ------------------------------123
Thyme-lemon Garlic Mushrooms ---------------125

Desserts -- 127
Mock Cinnabon -----------------------------------127
Baked Cream Cheese -----------------------------128
Fried Honey Banana -----------------------------130
Black Olives with Cheddar ----------------------132
White Chocolate Fat Bomb ----------------------133
Baby Greens with Grapefruit and Red Onion -134
Instant Pot Chocolate Fondue -------------------136
Chocolate Almond Keto Fat Bomb --------------138
Coconut Avocado Mousse ------------------------139
Nut Free Keto Brownie --------------------------140
Secret Ingredient Chocolate Mousse -----------142

Berries with Chocolate Ganache ---------------- *144*

Conclusion --- 145

Do You Like My Book & Approach To Publishing? -- 146

1: First, I'd Love It If You Leave a Review of This Book on Amazon. -------------------------------- *146*

2: Check Out My Other Keto Diet Books ------- *146*

3: Let's Get In Touch ---------------------------- *148*

4: Grab Some Freebies On Your Way Out; Giving Is Receiving, Right? ------------------------------ *148*

5: Suggest Topics That You'd Love Me To Cover To Increase Your Knowledge Bank. ------------ *149*

PSS: Let Me Also Help You Save Some Money! -- 150

PS:

I have special interest in the Ketogenic diet. My wife has been following the Ketogenic diet and I can honestly say that the journey has been amazing. The diet works. And this is why I have committed to writing and publishing as many of the Ketogenic diet books as possible to give readers different options as far as the Ketogenic diet is concerned.

For instance, I have Ketogenic diet books exclusively dedicated for:

- Breakfast
- Main Meals
- Snacks
- Desserts
- Appetizers
- Soups
- Vegetarians
- Crockpot/slow cooker users
- Instant pot users
- Air fryer users
- People who are on the Paleo diet
- People who are following intermittent fasting

- People who are following carb cycling

And much more.

You can check out my [Ketogenic Diet Books fan page shop](#) for more of the books, as I continue publishing more and more. If you want me to add your category of the Ketogenic diet books that I have published so far, make sure to send me a message. I will do the heavy lifting for you and get back to you with a book that you will love.

You could also subscribe to my newsletter to receive updates whenever I have something new: http://bit.ly/2Cketodietfanton.

Before we start discussing the different recipes you can prepare using 7 ingredients or less and in less than 30 minutes, let's start by building our understanding of what a Ketogenic diet is all about for the sake of complete beginners or those looking for a refresher.

If you want the recipes only, you can skip to the part with recipes.

A Comprehensive Overview of the Ketogenic Diet

What is Keto Diet?

Ketogenic diet is simply a diet that is very low in carbohydrates, high in fat, and moderate in protein.

I know this goes against all dieting knowledge you have gathered over the years, which says we should make sure to take high amounts of carbohydrates, moderate amounts of proteins and minimal amounts of fats but if you ask me, our intake of high amounts of carbs is perhaps the reason why we are constantly gaining weight. About a third of the world's population is overweight or obese. This is clearly sad because being overweight or obese exposes us to all manner of health risks some of which include type II diabetes, hypertension, heart disease, and much more. Think of the current prevalence of obesity as a ticking time bomb for a third of the world's population and you will get a good feel of just why this is saddening. If it were something like HIV/AIDs, flu and any other disease, there would be a public outcry but we somewhat seem to have gotten used to the problem.

The Ketogenic diet seeks to reverse this problem by recommending significant reduction of carb intake coupled with intake of high amounts of fats and moderate amounts of proteins. The reason for doing that is to push the body into a metabolic state referred to as ketosis. You do this by starving the body of carbohydrates so that it can make the most use of the available dietary fat (what you take in your diet) and body fat, which the body burns when the available dietary fat is not enough to fuel its different processes.

I know you are wondering; so how much is low, when it comes to the amount of carbohydrates that you should take while on this diet? Well, it is recommended that you don't exceed 50grams of carbohydrates per day (the lower the better) in order to effectively and swiftly push the body into ketosis. All you do now is to pair the less than 50grams of carbohydrates with 0.7-1 gram of protein for every pound of body weight as well and make sure 60-70% of your calories intake constitute healthy fats.

So how does this end up causing weight loss? What's the explanation behind the process of ketosis?

Well, in order to understand ketosis, it is important that you understand one very important thing; carbohydrates, not fats make us fat. Your understanding of how that comes about is the first step to understanding how ketosis comes to reverse this.

Ketogenic Diet

When you eat, the body spends the next few hours breaking down the food you've eaten into easy to digest molecules. More precisely, it breaks down carbohydrates, fats and proteins into glucose, fatty acids and amino acids respectively. This process takes place at different speeds with carbohydrates being the fastest to break down followed by fats and then proteins. So when you eat lots of carbohydrates, as most of us do owing to the fact that we follow the conventional American diet, our body breaks down the available carbohydrates swiftly then absorbs the glucose into the bloodstream where it is to be transported to different parts of the body. For the absorption of glucose into cells to take place, your body relies on a hormone known as insulin to make that happen. It (insulin) does that by signaling the insulin receptors that all cells have. These receptors are triggered to tell the cells to 'open up' to take glucose. As long as there is glucose in the bloodstream, insulin keeps signaling the receptors to keep the 'doors' to the cells open so that as much of it can be absorbed as possible. This is important because high blood glucose concentrations can be harmful to the cells if this persists as they create an acidic environment. So even if the cells have had enough of the glucose, insulin keeps sending signals to the cells for them to take in glucose to clear any excess from the bloodstream to get the glucose to the base level. The body already has a mechanism for storing this excess glucose though; the liver converts the excess into glycogen, which is then stored in the liver and muscle cells. This process takes place with the help of insulin and is meant to salvage the situation by providing a temporary storage area for glucose while it awaits to be used during periods when you engage in strenuous physical activity or when you fast. As you may have guessed, this storage is very limited, as it can only take up to about 2000kcal of energy so if this limit is reached, the body has to find an alternative to store the excess glucose. The body considers this a long term storage need because if glycogen stores are full, they can take the body several days before they can be exhausted e.g. during times of extended fasting/starvation. This means if the body has enough for immediate use, it would be okay if it stored some of the glucose for use in a distant future. For this to be possible, with the help of insulin, the liver converts the excess glucose into fatty acids and glycerol, which are then transported to different fat stores around the body for storage e.g. under the skin, around different organs etc. If this takes place multiple times and over a long period, this is how you gain weight (become fat).

The Ketogenic diet seeks to reverse that by starving the body of the dietary molecule that ends up being converted into fat i.e. glucose, something that brings about a reverse of the process of storing fat.

How does that happen, you may ask? Let me explain that:

When you limit how much carb you take significantly, the body won't have enough glucose to sustain its different processes using glucose, leave alone have some left for storage. This means along with using dietary carbohydrates for energy, the body will be forced to use the available sources of energy. In that case, with reduced carb intake, your body will start using up all the available glucose for energy. This in turn comes with reduced insulin levels (insulin won't have much work for it to do since insulin is produced in response to rising blood glucose levels) something that prompts the body to secrete another hormone to counter the effects of reduced insulin levels. This hormone is known as glucagon and is produced by the pancreas (which also produces insulin). The work of glucagon is to signal the liver to initiate the process of metabolizing any available glycogen to glucose after which the body uses it just like dietary glucose. Other hormones like the human growth hormone are also produced. All these i.e. reduced insulin levels paired with more glucagon and the human growth hormone being availed result to a reversal of everything that insulin was doing. This includes releasing the stored fats into the bloodstream for transportation to the liver where they are metabolized into fatty acids and glycerol. These then go through several metabolic processes, which ultimately produce energy molecules known as ketones. Ketones are the equivalent of glucose in many ways with the major one being the fact that unlike fatty acids, they are water soluble and can therefore cross the blood brain barrier hence making them capable of fueling up to 70% of the brain processes. The process through which ketones are produced is referred to what is referred to as ketosis. Ketosis therefore is a metabolic process through which the body relies on ketones for energy as opposed to relying on glucose for energy. Your concentration of ketones keeps rising with time i.e. the more you get accustomed to living with very little amount of carbs. It (the concentration) can go to what is referred to as optimal ketosis, a state where the body is at an optimal fat burning fat at 1.0mmol/L and 3.0mmol/L.

Owing to the huge amounts of fat available (and considering that a gram of fat has more than double the amount of energy in amino acids and glucose), this essentially means you have huge amounts of 'fuel' to burn for your body's energy. And as that happens, it comes with a number of effects on the body, which manifest as benefits. Let's discuss some of these in the next chapter.

Benefits of Ketogenic Diet

Following a Ketogenic diet can bring you a number of benefits some of which we will discuss in this chapter.

1. Facilitate weight loss

As you should be aware by now, there is a direct link between carb intake and weight or fat gain. The Ketogenic diet helps reverse this by through the process of ketosis. When you are in ketosis, the body is using fats heavily to produce the needed ketones to meet the body's energy needs during times of depleted carbohydrate levels.

Other than the ketosis process, a Keto diet can help you lose weight because of several reasons:

First, as opposed to processed snacks and other high carbohydrate foods, eating fat makes you eat less due to the effective satiating effect it induces on your metabolism. When you eat foods like cheese, fatty fish, avocado and nuts, the fat content gets into the intestines and triggers release of hormones. Such hormones among them the cholecystokinin and Peptide YY help to control satiety and appetite and can make you feel fuller for longer. The satiating effect of fat is linked to its complexity in chemical composition that demands for a longer time to digest and extra energy for breakdown. A scientific study found out polyunsaturated fats, commonly referred to as "PUFAs", have the ability to trigger fullness to a bigger extent than meals with lower fatty acids.

Eating a high fat diet can also help you stick to your diet plan and in turn burn extra fat or lose weight.

Secondly, fat speeds up the rate of metabolism compared to a low-fat or high carb diet due to its link with fat burning hormones called adipokines. Hormones such as adiponectin are formed from fat cells and their work is to boost the rate at which fats are metabolized. To further explain the importance of eating fats, a study found out that eating healthier fat can help speed up metabolism and reduce storage of visceral or belly fat. Findings in this study showed that people who consumed high-fat foods burned 300 more calories daily compared to the low-fat group. Better still, the high-fat group had a normal amount of blood insulin and was less likely to develop related diabetic condition. The high fat group fed on 60 percent fats, 30 percent proteins and only 10 percent carbs while the low-fat group consumed 60 percent carbs, 20 percent fats and 20 percent proteins.

In addition, fat acts as a solvent for fat-soluble nutrients such as vitamin A, D, E, and K. The body needs to absorb such nutrients to facilitate various metabolic functions, and deficiency of these nutrients can be detrimental. Lack of essential minerals and vitamins can lead to problems such as blood clots, blindness, brittle bones, blood clots among others. For weight loss, you need vitamin D, as it helps metabolize body fat from regions such as the abdomen.

2. Help Monitor Blood Sugar

As stated earlier, carb foods are digested into glucose, and this makes the level of blood glucose to rise. Afterwards, insulin hormone, which is tasked with helping body cells absorb glucose from the blood stream, is secreted. Normally, high blood sugar shouldn't be a major problem since it takes a few hours for glucose to get absorbed into cells and to be depleted. But in exceptional cases, you might be suffering from insulin related complications such as resistance to insulin. This resistance is a condition where body cells stop being as responsive to insulin as a result of the excessive bombardment by insulin to take up glucose (when you have consistently high levels of glucose in the bloodstream as a result of taking lots of carb).

With insulin resistance, your blood would still have high sugar levels despite the elevated insulin levels, a condition that can damage body cells. For instance, elevated sugar levels can damage insulin-producing beta cells of your pancreas and other major blood vessels. Once the beta cells in the pancreas are damaged, you cannot produce sufficient or any insulin and you're said to be suffering from type II diabetes.

In addition to blood glucose control, insulin hormone also has an effect on metabolism of fatty acids, in a process referred to as lipolysis. High insulin level means that the body focuses on breakdown of carbs for fuel and hence the fatty acids or stored glycerol would remain intact in the adipose tissue. But by consuming low-carb Keto foods, you avoid rise in blood sugar that could make body cells fail to respond to insulin. Eating a low carb diet also means little or no insulin is secreted, as dietary fats require no insulin hormone to breakdown.

Actually, within 6 months of low-carb high fat diet, it's possible to reduce daily dosage of insulin by up to 50 percent according to a scientific study. This study has found out that around 95 percent of diabetics are able to abandon diabetes medication within 6 months of following Ketogenic diet. That's worthwhile don't you think?

In simplest terms, Ketogenic diet is very important for weight loss and can also be a life savior against metabolic diseases such as heart disease, diabetes or obesity. And just like other diets, there are specific foods to eat and those to ditch so as to achieve optimal ketosis or high rate of fats breakdown. The initial step into Ketogenic diet is to lower intake of carbs and focus more on healthy fats as well as lean healthy proteins from meat, eggs and dairy. However, excess intake of proteins can hinder ketosis process, as the excess protein is converted into glucose through a processed referred to as *gluconeogenesis*. The glucose converted from excess protein has potential to raise blood sugar level, which in turn increases your insulin levels and this cycle continues.

So how do you strike balance? First, ensure that your intake of carb revolves around 50 grams or less of carbs in a day. Then you should control protein intake to enable your metabolism to continue producing ketone bodies. Regulate this to just 0.7-1 gram of protein per pound of body weight to ensure the body obtains fuel just from ketone bodies formed from fatty foods. You should also eat more healthy fats and oils as fat can fight cravings and induce satiety. The higher the fat intake, the lesser proteins and carbs you consume;

which drops down insulin level and get you into optimal ketosis.

With that in mind, let's see what you should eat in Keto diet:

What To Eat On Keto

There are different classes of foods that constitute this diet; but these have to be taken in the right proportion to achieve the benefits of a Ketogenic diet. What you should know is that the bulk of Ketogenic diet is healthy fats and oils as well as lean proteins. So which foods you should you eat?

1. Fats and Oils

Though these form the bulk of Keto diet, you should be aware that not all fats are good and healthy for you. Actually, saturated fats like hydrogenated oils and Trans fatty acids can trigger cardiovascular diseases such as the heart disease. The most recommended fats to reach for are omega 3 fatty oils, unsaturated and mono-saturated fats. These types of fats are preferred because they have a stable chemical structure and don't cause inflammatory diseases.

Such fats include:

- Ghee

- Avocado and avocado oil

- Mayonnaise, sugar free

- Beef tallow

- Macadamia oil

- Coconut butter

- Almond oil

- Butter
- Duck fat, organic
- Olives and olive oil
- Coconut oil and coconut Butter
- Chicken fat
- Organic red palm oil
- Beef tallow, grass fed
- Duck fat
- Non hydrogenated lard
- Peanut butter, unsweetened
- Seed and nut oils like sesame oil or flaxseed oil

2. Veggies

These should form a considerable part of your diet, as they are rich source for vitamins that helps your immune system to fight diseases. In Keto diet, choose the leafy greens as these are high in nutrients and low on carbohydrates. Together with the dark leafy greens, here's complete list of veggies that you can choose from:

- Scallions
- Collard greens
- Broccoli

Ketogenic Diet

- Cauliflower
- Alfalfa Sprouts
- Bib lettuce
- Water chestnuts
- Turnips
- Celery
- Arugula
- Jalapeno peppers
- Spinach
- Kale
- Dill pickles
- Leeks
- Cabbage
- Romaine
- Cauliflower
- Cucumbers
- Asparagus
- Shallots
- Brussels sprouts

- Onion
- Garlic
- Artichoke hearts
- Beet Greens
- Bamboo Shoots
- Lettuces and salad greens
- Cabbage
- Swiss chard
- Radishes
- Chard
- Mushrooms

3. Proteins

A sufficient protein intake facilitates general growth as well as repair of worn out cells. But as stated before, you must moderate proteins intake to inhibit conversion of amino acids into glucose, as this can hinder the metabolism of stored fat. Eat lean proteins from pastured animals, as these are less likely to be contaminated with pesticides and other chemicals.

Eat these in moderation:

- Steak

- Ham
- Crab
- Salmon
- Cod
- Eggs
- Ground beef
- Pork Loin, Chops & Steaks
- Bacon
- Sausages
- Tilapia
- Shrimp
- Tuna
- Offal, grass-fed
- Chicken breasts and thighs
- Pork/Beef/Lamb roasts

4. Nuts & Seeds

Both seeds and nuts can be a healthier snack option since Keto diet bans consumption of wheat, baked goods and most pre-packaged or processed snacks.

Since these contain carb too, moderate intake to just a handful a day. Eat these:

- Brazil nuts
- Flax seeds
- Pine Nuts
- Sunflowers seeds
- Flaxseed
- Sesame seeds
- Pumpkin seeds
- Walnuts
- Almonds
- Pistachios
- Hazelnuts
- Macadamias
- Hemp Seeds
- Pecans
- Hazelnuts

5. Fruits

As opposed to veggies, most fruits are high in fructose and sugars hence only a few are recommended. More precisely, you can eat 2-3 servings daily provided you choose low-carb version that has no added sugars or sauces.

Reach for berries and other fruits like:

- Avocado
- Strawberries
- Blackberries
- Coconut
- Blueberries
- Cranberries
- Olives
- Rhubarb
- Raspberries

6. Beverages

Most drinks such as soft drinks, alcohol and processed dairy are rich in carbs and processed sugars. However, you can drink a few unsweetened beverages such as:

- Lemon juice
- Almond milk
- Coconut milk
- Water

- Herbal tea
- Soy milk
- Clear broth, bone broth
- Decaf tea
- Flavored seltzer water
- Lime juice
- Decaf coffee

7. Dairy products

Milk and other processed dairy products contain high content of lactose, a type of sugar that can alter blood-sugar levels. If you want to drink milk, fermented milk products have less lactose since the bacteria used to ferment consumes up all the lactose.

Choose the following products:

- Sour cream, full fat
- Cream cheese
- Full fat cottage cheese
- Heavy whipping cream
- Mascarpone cheese
- Hard and soft cheese
- Full-fat cheese

- Whole milk yogurt, unsweetened

8. Condiments and sweeteners

Keto diet restricts use of artificial sweeteners but you can adopt few sweeteners like honey, stevia or maple syrup to sweeten foods. Be aware that artificially sweetened snacks and salty foods aren't Keto friendly and thus you should do away with them. Choose your condiments from these foods:

- Extra dark chocolate
- Cocoa and carob powder
- Ketchup, sugar-free
- Tomato puree
- mints, sugar-free
- Arrowroot powder
- Stevia
- Erythritol
- Chewing gums

Foods to Avoid

Apart from moderating intake of nuts, seeds, starchy veggies and high carb fruits; there are foods that you should do away with completely. These include grains, refined sugars, corns and legumes.

Let's see why:

1. Sugary foods

Eating sugars and processed carbs can disrupt blood sugar level and spike the level of insulin hormone. A spike in insulin level is attributed to cravings and hunger; and can make you to end up overeating. Worse still, insulin controls the fat metabolism and unfortunately, the higher the amount of insulin secreted, the more the fat the body stores. With that knowledge, avoid these sugars:

- Glucose
- Fruit juice concentrates
- Brown rice syrup
- Honey and agave nectar
- Cane juice crystals
- Brown sugar
- Cane syrup
- Canned soups and stews

- Maple syrup
- Fructose
- Fruit syrup
- Malt syrup
- Coconut sugar
- Molasses
- Barley malt and malt powder
- Cane sugar
- Sorghum
- Maltose
- Cane juice
- Rice syrup
- Date sugar
- Dextrose

2. Sugary beverages

These include drinks such as juices from veggies and fruits, non-diet sodas as well as alcohol. Juices are made from concentrated sugar of the original fruit while non-diet sodas like corn syrup contain large amounts of fructose. Also, avoid most beers and alcohol products as these are made from high carb grains like barley.

Also avoid the following:

- Apple juice
- Beers
- Grape juice
- Orange juice
- Alcohol and mixers
- non-diet sodas
- Sweet or dessert wines
- juice from fruits
- Vodka
- Mango juice
- Strawberry juice
- Whiskey
- Rum
- Tequila
- Star-fruit juice

3. Grains and corn

Though very delicious and widely available, you should not eat wheat flour, pasta, pancakes, cookies and cakes. More precisely, avoid every food material that has grain in it, whether whole-grain, processed grains or whatever kind of grains you can come across. Be aware that corn can be used as a thickener or preservative in other products so remember to read a list of ingredients in products that you buy.

Avoid the following types of grains:

- Bread crumbs
- Pancakes
- Popcorn
- Cookies, Tarts
- Crackers
- Hot cereals
- Tortillas
- Oatmeal
- Corn chips
- Tamale Wrappers
- Cornmeal
- Polenta
- Grits
- Pasta
- Waffles

- Cereals
- High-Fructose Corn Syrup
- Pretzels
- Cakes
- Cold cereals
- English muffins
- Sandwiches
- Wheat thins
- Pancakes
- Cornbread
- Pies
- Breads rolls

4. Starchy tubers and veggies

Avoid starchy foods and tubers like squashes, potatoes, sweet potatoes and yams due to their high carb content. This also applies to their products such as potato chips, French fries and tater. Avoid these:

- Acorn squash
- Potatoes
- Sweet potatoes

- Beets
- Yam
- Butternut squash
- Okra
- Yucca

5. Legumes

Beans, lentils and peas are protein foods but on the other hand contain high starch content. To restrict carb intake to below 50 grams threshold, avoid all legumes such as the following:

- Snow peas
- Green beans
- Kidney beans
- Black beans
- Broad beans
- Lentils
- Sugar snap peas
- Garbanzo beans
- String beans
- Pinto beans

- White beans
- Lima beans
- Adzuki beans
- Soybeans
- Chickpeas
- Black-eyed peas
- Horse beans
- Navy beans
- Red beans
- Mesquite

While going Keto is healthy, it's a fact that doing away with your favorite foods such as baked goods, grains, soft drinks and fruit juice can be challenging at first. So if you find it hard to cut out these foods out of your diet all at once, try to gradually reduce the amount you consume until well adapted. It's easier to handle diet change in slow transitions over long term, and it can bring better results in terms of handling cravings. While that could be a very challenging undertaking, try adopting a step by step approach to achieve the many tangible benefits of the diet.

For starters, in Ketogenic diet, here are delicious and quick to prepare recipes to get you started:

Keto Recipes with 7 Ingredients or Less That You Can Prepare Within 30 Minutes

Breakfast Recipes

5-Ingredient Keto Mug Lasagna

Prep Time: 15 Minutes

Cook Time: 5 Minutes

Total Time: 20 Minutes

Calories: 270, Carbs: 3g, Protein: 6g, Fat: 27g

Serves: 1

Ingredients

Italian seasoning

3 tablespoons full-fat mozzarella, shredded

6-8 tablespoons full fat ricotta cheese

6-8 tablespoons marinara, sugar-free

1/3 zucchini, thinly sliced

Directions

1. Begin by slicing the zucchini into paper-thin rounds and then set aside.

2. Add a tablespoon of marinara sauce to a mug and spread it to cover the bottom part of the mug.

3. Now layer the sliced zucchini and spread a tablespoon of ricotta cheese on the top.

4. Repeat this entire process of layering until the mug is somehow full

5. Add in another layer of zucchini rounds and now top with mozzarella cheese.

6. Microwave the contents on high heat for about 4 to 5 minutes or until done.

7. Finally remove the microwave and then top with Italian seasoning if you like it.

Flaxseed Muffin in a Mug

Prep Time: 2 Minutes

Cook Time: 1 Minute

Total Time: 3 Minutes

Calories 283, Carbs 11.7g, Protein 11.8g, Fat 21.9g

Servings: 1 mug muffin

Ingredients

1 tablespoon erythirtol or 1-2 drops stevia

1/4 teaspoon ground cinnamon

1/2 teaspoon baking powder

1/4 cup flaxmeal

1 teaspoon vanilla extract

1 teaspoon extra virgin coconut oil, melted

1 egg

Directions

1. First, whisk the vanilla, oil and the egg together and set the mixture aside.

2. Stir in the dry ingredients such as the baking powder, flax meal, sugar-free sweetener and cinnamon.

3. Stir in optional add-ons such as chocolate chips and raspberries if you like it and then move to a 2.5 inch high mug.

4. Microwave the contents for 1 minute 30 seconds on high heat then serve.

Sugar-Free Lemon Mug Cake

Prep Time: 3 minutes

Cook Time: 1 minute

Total Time: 4 minutes

Calories 233, Carbs 11g, Protein 8g, Fat 17g

Servings: 1

Ingredients

Pinch salt

1/4 teaspoon baking powder

2 tablespoons coconut flour

1/2 teaspoon lemon liquid stevia

2 tablespoons heavy cream

2 tablespoons lemon juice

1 egg

Directions

1. Begin by whisking the egg with cream, lemon juice and stevia in a bowl.

2. Then stir in baking powder, salt and coconut flour.

3. At this point, pour in the batter in a 7-ounce ramekin and then microwave until a toothpick inserted in the center of the

mug comes out clean. This should be in about 30 to 60 seconds.

4. Serve the cake topped with whipped cream if you like it.

Vanilla Keto Mug Cake

Prep Time: 5 minutes

Cook Time: 5 minutes

Total Time: 10 minutes

Calories 334, Carbs 7.9g, Protein 11.8g, Fat 28.6g

Serves 1

Ingredients

1 tablespoon extra-virgin coconut oil or butter, melted

1 large egg, free-range or organic

2 tablespoons Erythritol or Swerve

1/8 teaspoons baking soda

1/2 teaspoons sugar-free vanilla extract or 1/4 teaspoons vanilla bean powder

1 heaping tablespoons coconut flour

2 heaping tablespoons almond flour

Optional

3-5 drops liquid stevia

2 tablespoons coconut milk, full-fat yogurt or whipped cream,

A pinch of cinnamon

Directions

1. Put all the dry ingredients in a ramekin or mug and mix well to incorporate.

2. Add in the egg, stevia along with coconut oil. Mix the contents using a fork and then microwave for 70 to 90 seconds on high heat.

3. In case you don't have a microwave, you can also cook in a preheated oven at 350 degrees F. Cook until the cake cooked in the center or for about 12 to 15 minutes.

Optional:

4. Once cooked through, top with full-fat yoghurt, creamed coconut milk or whipped cream if you like it.

One-Minute Keto Mug Bread

Prep Time: 1 minute

Cook Time: 1 minute

Total Time: 2 minutes

Calories 277, Carbs 2.0g, Protein 9.98g, Fat 25.54g

Servings: 1

Ingredients

1 tablespoon olive oil

1 egg

1/2 teaspoon baking powder

4 tablespoons almond meal/flour

Pinch of salt

Directions

1. Mix together all the ingredients in a mug using a fork until well incorporated.

2. Once very wet, microwave the batter on high for about 60 seconds. Tap the top of the mug bread to ensure it's cooked through and if not done, microwave for additional 20 to 30 seconds.

3. At this point, turn the mug upside down to remove the bread, and allow it to cool.

4. Slice and serve, or instead toast it for crispier texture. You can serve it alone or as a sandwich bun.

Ketogenic Cloud Eggs

Prep Time: 15 minutes

Cook Time: 5 minutes

Total Time: 20 minutes

Calories 241, Carbs 9.7g, Protein 22.9g, Fat 12g

Serves 4

Ingredients

1/2 pounds deli ham, chopped

1 cup Parmesan, freshly grated

Black pepper, freshly ground

Kosher salt

8 large eggs

Fresh chives, finely chopped

Directions

1. First, preheat your oven to 450 degrees and then line a baking sheet using a parchment paper.

2. Now separate the egg yolks from the whites, and put the yolks in a small bowl and egg whites in a large bowl.

3. Season the whites with some pepper and salt. Then whisk the egg whites using a hand mixer or a whisk. Beat until it starts forming stiff peaks.

4. Now fold in the cheese, ham and the chives. Next, make 4 mounds using the egg whites on a baking sheet and then indent the centers of each to resemble nests.

5. Then bake the mounds for around 3 minutes, or until somehow golden.

6. At this point, add an egg yolk in the middle of egg white cloud. Season with pepper and salt and then bake for about 3 minutes. Once the egg yolks are set, serve.

Bell Pepper Eggs

Prep Time: 5 minutes

Cook Time: 15 minutes

Total Time: 20 minutes

Calories 268, Carb 4.19g, Protein 18.45g, Fat 19.37g

Serves 3

Ingredients

2 tablespoons parsley, chopped

2 tablespoons chives, chopped

Black peppers, freshly ground

Kosher salt

6 eggs

1 bell pepper, sliced into ¼ inch rings

Directions

1. Over medium heat, heat a nonstick skillet and then lightly grease it with some cooking spray.

2. In the skillet, add in bell pepper ring and sauté the veggies for about 2 minutes.

3. Flip the red pepper and then crack an egg in the middle of it. Season the ring with sufficient amount of pepper and salt.

4. Then cook the mixture until the egg is done, in about 2 to 4 minutes. Repeat the process with the rest of the eggs.

5. Finally garnish with chopped parsley and a handful of chives.

Bacon Egg Muffin Cups

Prep Time: 10 minutes

Cook Time: 10 minutes

Total Time: 20 minutes

Calories 283, Carbs 6.87g, Protein 14.53g, Fat 21.57g

Serves: 12

Ingredients

12 tablespoons shredded parmesan cheese

12 slices of bacon

12 eggs

6 slices of keto friendly bread (you can use One-Minute Keto Mug Bread that we prepared earlier)

Directions

1. Preheat the oven to about 400 degrees F.

2. On medium-high heat, heat a skillet until hot and then cook the bacon for 4-5 minutes.

3. Meanwhile, cut 2 circles from each bread slice, preferably using a cookie cutter. (Reserve the extra bread or feed it to the birds if you like it.)

4. Spray the muffin tin with cooking spray, and then lay a circle of bread into each cup's bottom-most part. Then wrap around the edge of every muffin cup with bacon.

5. Now sprinkle the cheese on the bread slices. Next, crack one egg carefully into each cup or crack it into a bowl first and slide into a muffin cup.

6. Bake the cups until the egg whites get set and the yolk is well cooked, or for around 10-15 minutes.

7. Finally top the pancakes with some fresh fruits and enjoy.

Keto Mushroom Omelet

Prep Time: 5 minutes

Cook Time: 15 minutes

Total Time: 20 minutes

Calories 510, Fat 43g, Carbs 5.8g, Protein 25g

Serves 1

Ingredients

3 mushrooms

1/5 yellow onion

30g shredded cheese

30g butter

3 eggs

Salt

Pepper

Directions

1. In a mixing bowl, crack in the eggs and then season with salt and pepper. Whisk using a fork to obtain a smooth and frothy consistency.

2. Add in other spices and additional salt if need be. Now melt butter in a pan, and pour in the egg in the frying pan as soon as the butter melts.

3. Cook until the omelet gets cooked and is hard but with some parts of raw egg remaining on top.

4. At this point, sprinkle with mushrooms, cheese and onions if you like.

5. Ease around the edges of the omelet using a spatula and now fold it over in half.

6. As soon as the omelet begins to brown underneath, remove the frying pan from heat and set the hot omelet on a plate to serve.

7. You can top with green salad and vinaigrette dressing on top if you like.

Frittata with Tomatoes and Cheese

Prep Time: 10 minutes

Cook Time: 5 minutes

Total Time: 15 minutes

Calories 435, *Carbs 7.4g, Protein 26.7g, Fat 32.6 g*

Serves 2

Ingredients

2 tablespoon herbs, freshly chopped

2/3 cup cherry tomatoes, halved

1 tablespoon ghee

2/3 cup soft cheese like feta, crumbled

½ medium white onion

6 large eggs, free-range or organic

Black pepper, freshly ground and sea salt

Directions

1. Preheat your oven to 400 degrees F. Meanwhile, peel and slice the onion.

2. On a pan greased with ghee, cook the onion until slightly browned.

3. In a bowl, crack the eggs and then season with pepper and salt. Add chopped herbs such as chives and mix well.

4. Pour in the eggs in the browned onion and cook until the edges turn opaque.

5. Top with halved cherry tomatoes and crumbled cheese. Put under a broiler and cook until the top is cooked.

6. After 5-7 minutes, remove from the oven and allow to cool. Serve and enjoy.

Fast Fat Herbed Omelet

Prep Time: 10 minutes

Cook Time: 5 minutes

Total Time: 15 minutes

Calories 719, carbs: 7.2g, Protein: 30.1g, Fat: 63.3g

Serves 4

Ingredients

1 slice of bacon crisped up (30g /1 oz.)

1/2 small avocado around 50g

2 tablespoons ghee, butter or coconut oil

1/2 tablespoon oregano, freshly chopped

1 tablespoon basil, freshly chopped

1/2 cup grated Parmesan cheese

2 large eggs, free-range or organic

Directions

1. Grate the cheese and set aside.

2. Then crack the eggs into a medium bowl, and add in grated Parmesan cheese and chopped herbs such as oregano and basil. You can also use spring onion, parsley or chives in place of herbs.

3. Grease a skillet with coconut oil, ghee or butter then heat it over medium high heat. Once hot, pour in the egg mixture and reduce the heat to low.

4. Bring in the omelet from the sides towards the center using a spatula for about 30 seconds to ensure even cooking.

5. Once the tops are firm, flip to cook the other side for around 30 seconds. If need be, you can fold the omelet in half and cook for additional 30-60 seconds.

6. Once done, put the omelet on a serving plate then top with sliced avocado and crisped up bacon.

Bacon and Brie Frittata

Prep Time: 5 minutes

Cook Time: 20 minutes

Total Time: 25 minutes

Calories 327, Carbs 1.91g, Protein: 16.68g, Fat: 25.93g

Serves 10-inch frittata

Ingredients

1/2 teaspoon pepper

1/2 teaspoon salt

2 cloves garlic, minced

1/2 cup whipping cream

8 large eggs

8 slices bacon, chopped

4 ounces brie, sliced thin

Directions

1. Cook the bacon in a 10-inch sauté pan over medium heat.

2. Once crisp, remove from heat using a slotted spoon and set on a towel-lined plate.

3. Set aside the skillet along with 2 tablespoon of bacon grease.

4. Whisk together two-thirds of the cooked bacon with eggs, cream, pepper, salt and garlic in a large bowl.

5. Heat the skillet over medium low heat and then swirl the reserved bacon grease to coat the bottoms and sides.

6. In the skillet, pour the egg mixture and cook until the edges are set and the center is loose; undisturbed. This should take about 10 minutes.

7. Meanwhile, heat a broiler and then put an oven rack on the second highest setting in the oven.

8. Put the slices of brie on the frittata and sprinkle with reserved bacon. Broil until it's puffed and golden.

9. After around 5 minutes, remove from heat and cool.

Lunches

Orange and Sage Glazed Duck Breast

Prep Time: 5 minutes

Cook Time: 20 minutes

Total Time: 25 minutes

Calories 798, Carbs 1g, Protein 36g, Fat 71g

Serves 4

Ingredients

1 tablespoon swerve or other natural sweetener

1 tablespoon heavy cream

1 cup spinach

2 tablespoons butter

16 ounces ducks breast

1/2 teaspoons orange extract

1/4 teaspoon sage

Directions

1. First score the duck skin from the duck breast and then season with pepper and salt.

2. Add butter into a pan over medium-low heat and then lower the heat for the butter to lightly brown.

3. Once browned, add orange extract and sage and continue cooking until the butter is deep amber colored.

4. Into a separate pan, put the breast and then heat over medium high for few minutes. Flip the meat occasionally until you achieve a crisp skin.

5. Now add heavy cream to the mixture and stir to incorporate. Pour the cream sage butter mixture onto the duck breast and allow to coat.

6. Cook the breast for a few more minutes before serving. Then wilt some spinach in the pan to prepare a sauce if you like.

7. If need be, allow the duck to rest for 2 to 3 minutes, and finally slice it and put it on top of the spinach with the sauce.

10-Minute Instant Pot Salmon

Prep Time: 5 minutes

Cook Time: 5 minutes

Total Time: 10 minutes

Calories 406, Carbs 2.6g, Protein 65.6g, Fat 15.32g

Serves: 4

Ingredients

1/4 teaspoon black pepper, ground

1/4 teaspoon salt

1 tablespoon butter, unsalted

1 bunch dill weed, fresh

4 fillets salmon

3/4 cup water

3 medium lemon

Directions

1. Put the water and juiced lemon in the bottom of the cooking pot then insert the steamer insert.

2. Put the salmon fillets on the steamer insert, sprinkle some dill on top of the salmon, then put a fresh lemon on each of the fillets.

3. Secure the lid in place and now set the timer to about 5 minutes.

4. As soon as the timer beeps, quick release the steam and then careful open the lid.

5. Serve the fish with lemon, green beans, extra dill and butter.

Ahi Tuna Poke Recipe

Prep Time: 10 minutes

Cook Time: 0 minute

Total Time: 10 minutes

380 Calories, Carbs 3.1g, Protein 29.5g, Fat 26.5g

Serves 2

Ingredients

1/2 head Boston or butter lettuce, leaves separated

1 tablespoon black sesame seeds

3 tablespoons fresh cilantro, chopped

1/2 medium avocado, diced fine

1 tablespoon soy sauce

2 tablespoons sesame oil

8 ounces ahi tuna, boneless

Optional

Lime wedges (to serve)

Pinch salt

Directions

1. Begin by dicing the ahi tuna into small-sized cubes and then put them in a medium bowl.

2. Toss in pinch of salt, soy sauce and sesame oil and then add in sesame seeds, cilantro and avocado. Toss until well blended.

3. Now spoon the ahi tuna poke into lettuce cups and serve with some lime wedges if you like it.

Shake and Bake Pork Chop

Prep Time 0 minutes

Cook Time 30 minutes

Total Time: 30 minutes

Calories 350, Carbs 2g, Protein 51.5g, Fat 14g

Serves 6

Ingredients

1/4 teaspoon dried oregano

1/4 teaspoon onion powder

1/4 teaspoon garlic powder

1/2 teaspoon salt

1/2 teaspoon paprika

1/2 tablespoon psyllium husk powder

6 (6-ounce) boneless pork loin chops

Directions

1. Heat the oven to 350 degrees F. Meanwhile, line a baking sheet using a parchment paper and set aside.

2. Now rinse the pork chops in cool water before removing and then pat drying them.

3. Then mix together the spices and psyllium husk powder in a zippered freezer bag.

4. Add in the chops one by one and then shake well to coat, and put the chops on the prepared baking sheet.

5. At this point, bake until the internal temperature is at 145 degrees F or for about 30 minutes

6. Serve the dish while the pork chops are still hot.

Chili Roasted Chicken Thighs

Prep Time: 5 Minutes

Cook Time 15 minutes

Total Time: 20 minutes

Calories 237, Carbs 0g, Protein 29.42g, Fat 12.35g

Serves: 4

Ingredients

1 tablespoon chili powder

2 pounds boneless chicken thighs

Lime wedges for serving

Fresh cilantro for garnish

Directions

1. First heat the oven to 375 degrees F.

2. To a sheet pan, add in the chicken and then drizzle the meat with olive oil. Turn it around to coat in oil.

2. Season the chicken with salt, chili powder and pepper and now roast the chicken for 15 minutes.

3. Once cooked through, remove the meat from the heat and sprinkle with cilantro. Serve with lime wedges if you like.

Garlic Ghee Pan-Fried Cod

Prep Time: 3 Minutes

Cook Time: 10 minutes

Total Time: 13 minutes

Calories: 160, Carbs: 1g, Protein: 21g, Fat: 7g

Serves: 4

Ingredients

6 cloves of garlic, minced

3 tablespoons ghee

4 cod fillets (approx. 0.3 pounds each)

Salt to taste

1 tablespoon garlic powder

Directions

1. In a frying pan, melt the ghee then add in minced garlic.

2. Put the cod fillets into the oiled pan and cook on medium to high heat until cooked through. Then season with garlic powder and salt.

3. Once the fish is white in color and the white color creeps halfway up the side, flip it and then season with minced garlic.

4. Continue cooking until the entire filet turns solid white or it flakes easily.

5. Serve the fish with ghee from the pan and some garlic.

Prosciutto Melon Wrap-Ups

Prep Time: 5 minutes

Cook Time: 5 minutes

Total Time: 10 minutes

Calories 79, Carbs 11g, Protein 5g, Fat 2g

Serves: 4

Ingredients

2 fresh sprig mint, chopped

1 package ham, prosciutto, sliced

½ medium honeydew melon or cantaloupe, seeded

Directions

1. Slice a cantaloupe carefully into 1 inch wedges and then take out the rinds.

2. Use the prosciutto to wrap each of the cantaloupes and then use toothpicks to secure if necessary.

3. You can garnish with fresh mint, and then serve it at room temperature or when cooled.

Basil Spinach Salad

Prep Time: 10 minutes

Cook Time: 5 minutes

Total Time: 15 minutes

Calories 146, Carbs 15g, Protein 5g, Fat 7g

Serves 2

Ingredients

1/2cup basil, fresh, several sprigs

4 handfuls spinach

2 medium tomatoes, diced

½ medium onions, yellow, diced

1 tablespoon coconut oil

Directions

1. Begin by washing and preparing the veggies.

2. Over medium heat, heat a small skillet and then add in coconut oil when fully hot.

3. Now add in diced onions, and sauté the mixture until it turns soft and translucent. At this point, add in the tomatoes and then cook for 2 additional minutes.

4. Finally, add in basil and spinach to this pan and cook for another 1 minute, and then serve it warm.

Beef, Scallions and Red Bell Pepper Sauté

Prep Time: 10 minutes

Cook Time: 10 minutes

Total Time: 20 minutes

Calories 387.5, Carbs 6.9g, Protein 37.5g, Fat 22.9g

Serves 1

Ingredients

1/4 cup mozzarella cheese, shredded

1/2 cup sweet red peppers, chopped

1/4 cup scallions or spring onions, chopped

5 ounces of steak

Directions

1. Over medium-high heat, sauté beef cut into thin strips in a small skillet for about 1 to 2 minutes.

2. Then add red pepper and scallions then sauté the mixture for the pepper to soften and the beef to become brown.

3. Now add in pepper and salt to taste and drain the extra fat.

4. Put the meat mixture onto a place and sprinkle the cheese. Let the cheese to melt before serving.

Fresh Tuna Salad

Prep Time: 5 minutes

Cook Time: 0 minutes

Total Time: 5 minutes

Calories 245, Carbs 12.04g, Protein 34.63g, Fat 7.1g

Serves 1

Ingredients:

Fine sea salt to taste

1 tablespoon of ketchup, optional

1 tablespoon of mayo

1/4 of a small purple onion, chopped

1 Persian cucumber, diced

1 Roma tomato, diced

1 can of tuna, drained

Directions

1. Add all the ingredients in a medium size bowl and mix well.

2. Serve the salad with sliced cucumbers and chips made without any vegetable oil such as Jacksons Honest chips.

Goat Cheese & Spinach Salad

Prep Time: 10 minutes

Cook Time: 10 minutes

Total Time: 20 minutes

Calories 645, Carbs 9.8g, Protein 33.2 g, Fat 54.2g

Serves 2

Ingredients

½ cup flaked almonds, toasted

4 cups spinach, fresh

1 ½ cup hard goat cheese, grated

4 strawberries for garnish

4 tablespoons Raspberry Vinaigrette (recipe included)

Directions

1. Preheat the oven to 400 degree F. Use parchment paper cut in half to line a baking tray.

2. Onto the baking sheet, grate the goat cheese in the shape of two rough circles.

3. Place the cheese in the preheated oven and bake for 10 minutes. Once golden in color, remove from the oven and cool down.

4. Place a small bowl up-side down, and then lift the parchment paper off the tray. Now flip the cheese over the bowl. Press the edges lightly and allow to cool for about 5 minutes.

5. To make salad filling (i.e. Raspberry Vinaigrette), pat-dry washed spinach with paper towel and put it in the cheese bowls.

6. Toss with berry vinaigrette, and sprinkle with almond flakes, toasted. If desired, top with strawberry slices.

5-Minute Keto Sardines Salad

Prep Time: 5 minutes

Cook Time: 0 minutes

Total Time: 5 minutes

Calories: 400, Carbs: 2g, Protein: 30g, Fat: 34g

Serves 1

Ingredients

1 tablespoon lemon juice

1 tablespoon olive oil

1/10 pounds bacon or leftover meat, chopped small

1/4 pounds salad greens

1 can sardines in olive oil or brine, drained

Salt to taste

Directions

1. Toss the salad greens in lemon juice and olive oil. Add in the bacon or leftover meat and toss to combine.

2. Toss the mixture with drained fish and sprinkle with salt. Serve and enjoy.

Dinner

Rosemary Garlic Chicken Kabobs

Prep Time 15 minutes

Cook Time 15 minutes

Total Time 30 minutes

Calories 168, Carb 0.46g, Protein 20g, Fat 9.1g

Serves 8

Ingredients

Several grinds black pepper

1 teaspoon kosher salt

3 cloves garlic minced

2 tablespoons chopped fresh rosemary

1/4 cup olive oil

3 boneless-skinless chicken breasts cut in bite-size pieces

8 bamboo skewers

Directions

1. Begin by soaking the bamboo skewers for about 15 minutes to prevent any possible burning.

2. Mix together the rest of the ingredients in a bowl large enough to accommodate them. Stir the mixture so as to coat all sides of the meat.

3. Now divide the chicken chunks and then thread them on the skewers. Cover the assembled kabobs and keep then chilled until ready to grill them.

4. Meanwhile, preheat the grill to 375 degrees F and then grill the chicken for about 3 minutes on each side, or cook the chicken until well cooked through.

5. Serve and enjoy.

Low Carb Pork Medallions

Prep Time: 15 Minutes

Cook Time: 20 Minutes

Total Time: 35 Minutes

Calories 519, Carbs 7g, Protein 46g, Fat 36g

Serves 2

Ingredients

1/4 cup oil

3 medium shallots (chopped fine)

1 pounds pork tenderloin

Directions

Begin by slicing the pork into ½ inch thick "chops". Then chop the shallots and put them on a medium-sized plate.

2. Add some oil in a skillet or cast iron and heat it then press each piece of pork chop into the shallots on each side. Press firmly to help the shallots stick to the pork.

3. Now put the pork pieces with the shallots in the oil and cook until cooked through.

4. Serve the pork medallions with veggies and enjoy!

Pesto Chicken with Mozzarella Casserole

Prep Time: 5 Minutes

Cook Time: 25 Minutes

Total Time: 30 Minutes

Calories 451, Carbs 3g, Protein 38g, Fat 30g

Serves: 8

Ingredients

8 oz. mozzarella shredded

2 lb. of cooked chicken breasts, cubed

8 oz. mozzarella cubed

1/4-1/2 cup heavy cream

8 oz. cream cheese softened

1/4 cup pesto

Directions

1. Heat the oven to 400 degrees F. Meanwhile, spray a large casserole using some cooking spray.

2. Mix together pesto, cream cheese and the heavy cream in a bowl and mix until smooth. You should use a ½ cup of cream for thinner sauce or ¼ cup cream to make thicker sauce.

3. Add in the cubed mozzarella and the chicken, and move the mixture to a casserole dish. Next, sprinkle the shredded cheese on top.

4. At this point, bake the dish for around 25 minutes and then serve with mashed cauliflower, spinach or zoodles if you like.

Spinach and Bacon Salad

Prep Time: 10 minutes

Cook Time: 0 minutes

Total Time: 10 minutes

Calories 531, Carbs 6.2g, Protein 21.0g, Fat 47.44g

Serves 2

Ingredients

1/4 cup plain mayonnaise

1/2 medium red onion, thinly sliced,

6 pieces thick sliced bacon

2 eggs boiled, cooled and cut in half then sliced

8oz. organic baby spinach (rinsed and dried)

Directions

1. Cook the bacon and boil the eggs then allow them to cool.

2. Now wash, rinse and dry the spinach if you like it. Peel and slice the boiled eggs and then slice the cooked onions.

3. At this point, cut the bacon into small sizes and serve it in a big glass bowl with the spinach and mayonnaise.

4. If you like it, add extra ingredients and fold then gently together.

Instant Pot Steamed Crab Legs

Prep Time: 5 minutes

Cook Time: 3 minutes

Total Time: 8 minutes

Calories 187.4, Carbs 6.7g, Protein 13.7g, Fat 11.9g

Servings: 4

Ingredients

4 tablespoon butter, melted

¾ cup water

Lemon juice

2 lbs. frozen crab legs

Directions

1. Place the steamer basket into the instant pot then put the crab legs on it.

2. Add in water and lock the lid in place.

3. Then cook for 2 minutes on high pressure then quick release. The crab meat once cooked should be bright pink in color.

4. Combine juice with some melted butter then serve.

Garlic Butter Brazilian Steak

Prep Time 10 minutes

Cook Time 5 minutes

Total Time 15 minutes

Calories 416, Carbs 4.6g, Protein 31.2g, Fat 30g

Serves: 4

Ingredients:

1 tablespoon fresh flat-leaf parsley, chopped

2 ounces (4 tablespoons) unsalted butter

2 tablespoons canola oil or vegetable oil

Black pepper, freshly ground

1 1/2 pounds skirt steak, trimmed and cut into 4 pieces

Kosher salt

6 medium cloves garlic

Directions

1. Peel the garlic cloves and then mash them using the side of a knife. Sprinkle with some salt and then mice the clove.

2. Now pat the steak dry and season with salt and pepper on both sides. Over medium heat, heat oil in a 12-inch heavy-duty skillet.

3. Once the oil is shimmering hot, add in the seasoned steak and brown for about 2 to 3 minutes on each side.

4. Move the steak to a plate and let cool until you are done making the garlic butter.

5. Meanwhile, melt butter in an 8-inch skillet over low heat. Then add in garlic and cook for 4 minutes as you swirl the pan a number of times.

6. Once lightly golden, lightly salt and taste. You can now slice the steak and distribute among 4 plates. To serve, spoon garlic butter over the steak and sprinkle with chopped parsley.

Jalapeno Cheddar Burgers

Prep Time: 15 minutes

Cook Time: 15 minutes

Total Time: 30 minutes

Calories: 413, Carbs: 1g, Protein: 46g, Fat: 23g

Serves 4 burger patties

Ingredients

1 fresh jalapeno pepper, diced

1/4 teaspoon garlic powder

2 ounce cheddar cheese, shredded

4 tablespoons cream cheese

2 tablespoons onion, finely minced

28 oz. lean turkey or beef

Salt & pepper to taste

Rolls & Toppings as desired

Directions:

1. Begin by heating your oven to broil on high heat or a grill to medium heat.

2. Mix together garlic powder, cheddar cheese, cream cheese and the diced jalapeno in a small bowl.

3. Mix together minced onion, pepper, meat and salt and then cut the meat into 4 equal pieces.

4. Obtain ¼ of the cheddar cheese mixture and flatten it to make a pancake.

5. Once done, wrap the turkey or beef around the cheese and ensure the mixture is fully covered by the meat.

6. At this point, brush each of the burgers using a little amount of olive oil. Grill the burgers on medium heat until well cooked, or for 6 to 7 minutes.

7. To broil, just place the burgers on a foil-lined pan about 6 inches from the broiler. Broil until fully cooked, or for 5 to 6 minutes on each side. (Beef should reach an internal temperature of 160 degrees and 165 degrees for turkey.)

Easy Buffalo Wings

Prep Time: 10 minutes

Cook Time: 20 minutes

Total Time: 30 minutes

Calories 620, Carbs 2g, Protein 48g, Fat 46g

Serves 2

Ingredients

2 tablespoons butter

1/2 cup Frank's Red Hot Sauce

6 chicken wings (6 wingettes, 6 drumettes)

Paprika

Garlic powder

Pepper

Salt

Cayenne (optional)

Directions

1. Break the chicken meat into two pieces, the drumetets and wingettes while discarding the tips.

2. Pour a little amount of hot sauce over the meat, to lightly coat them.

2. Now season the wings and toss to coat. Turn the broiler to high and put the meat on the oven rack about 6 inches from the broiler.

3. Line a baking sheet using aluminum foil and then lay the wings while allowing enough space between them for easy roasting.

4. Bake for about 15 minutes then serve.

Baked Bacon Cheddar Meatballs

Prep Time: 10 minutes

Cook Time: 20 minutes

Total Time: 30 minutes

Calories 375, Carbs 12.39g, Protein 26.06g, Fat 23.26g

Serves: 4

Ingredients

½ teaspoon pepper

½ teaspoon kosher salt

1 large egg

½ cup Italian seasoned breadcrumbs

½ cup sharp cheddar cheese, shredded

¼ pound bacon, browned and crumbled

¾ pound ground beef

Directions:

1. First preheat your oven to around 375 degrees F. Use aluminum foil to line a baking sheet.

2. Mix together the ingredients into a large mixing bowl, and then stir together entirely. From the mixture, create 1-inch thin balls of meat and position on the coated baking sheet.

3. Bake the balls until they turn golden, for about 20-25 minutes. Remember to flip once.

4. To serve, top with barbecue sauce if desired.

Low carb Skillet Lasagna

Prep Time: 3 minutes

Cook Time: 10 minutes

Total Time: 13 minutes

Calories 595, Carbs 7.2g, Protein 43.2g, Fat 30.7g

Serves 4

Ingredients

1 teaspoon fresh oregano, chopped

1 cup shredded mozzarella cheese divided, about 4 ounces

4 slices thin roast chicken breast from deli counter

24 ounce jar no sugar added marinara sauce

2 teaspoons fine sea salt

1 pound ground beef, 80% lean

Directions

1. Brown the beef in a 10 inch cast iron skillet over medium high heat, while seasoning the meat with sea salt as it cooks.

2. Cook the beef for around 5 minutes or until cooked through. Keep breaking up the beef using a spatula as it cooks.

2. Add in the sauce, stir to blend then push half of the cooked beef off one side of the skillet.

3. Now put a layer of sliced chicken breast on the bottom of the cooking pan and top the meat with half cup of shredded cheese.

4. Then scoop the beef on top of left over bacon to create an even layer. Top with the reserved 1/2 cup of cheese and sprinkle with some oregano.

5. Cover the mixture and heat on low to fully melt the cheese.

Low-Carb Pesto Baked Sea Bass

Prep Time: 5 minutes

Cook Time: 10 minutes

Total Time: 15 minutes

Calories 423, Carbs 2.3g, Protein 29.3g, Fat 32.9g

Serves 2

Ingredients

4 tablespoons pesto

1 tablespoon fresh lemon juice

1 tablespoon ghee, butter or coconut oil

2 large sea bass fillets

Salt to taste

Directions

1. Preheat the oven to 400 degrees F. Put the sea bass with the skin facing down into a baking dish that is lined with baking paper.

2. Season the sea bass with salt and brush the tops using ghee. Then add in a squeeze of lemon and put in the oven.

3. Now bake for about 10 minutes or until cooked through. Remove from the oven and top each serving with pesto.

4. Return the dish in the oven and bake for additional 3 to 5 minutes.

5. Then remove from heat and allow to cool for around 5 minutes or so. Serve it hot topped with preferred veggies and garlic.

Bunless Low Carb Burger

Prep Time: 5 Minutes

Cook Time: 10 Minutes

Total Time: 15 Minutes

Calories: 531, Carbs 5g, Protein: 26g, Fat: 45g

Serves 3

Ingredients

Salt and pepper

1 tablespoon Mc. Cormicks Montreal Steak Seasoning

1 tablespoon Worcestershire sauce

1 pound ground beef

Optional

4 ounces sliced onion

2 tablespoons bacon drippings or olive oil

Directions

1. Clean the grate and preheat the grill.

2. Then break the beef and distribute the steak seasoning, the sauce and olive oil if using.

3. Blend the mixture using your hands to evenly distribute the seasoning and then form the contents into 3 balls.

4. Pat or press the mixture into patties or use a burger press if you have one. You can make a slight depression in the center to prevent the burger from puffing up in the middle.

5. To cook, oil the grate and the season the outside of the patties with some salt and pepper.

6. Now grill the patties until done or until somehow pink in the middle. Serve the burger with Keto-friendly extras to avoid adding up carbs.

7. In case you want to make some caramelized onions, first slice the onions and then heat oil in a small pan over medium low-heat

8. Once hot, add in the sliced onions and sauté until well softened. Add in a little sweetener, erythritol.

9. Cook the onions until beginning to caramelize or brown, or for about 10 minutes.

Snacks

Cucumber Spinach Smoothie

Prep Time: 5 minutes

Cook Time: 0 minutes

Total Time: 5 minutes

Calories 330, Carbs 5.29g, Protein 10.14g, Fats 32.34g

Serves 1

Ingredients

1-2 tablespoon MCT oil

1/4 teaspoon xanthan gum

12 drops liquid stevia

1 cup coconut milk

7 ice cubes

2.5 oz. cucumber, peeled and cubed

2 handfuls spinach

Directions

1. Toss 2 handfuls of spinach into a blender then add in MCT oil, xanthan gum, stevia, coconut milk and the ice cubes.

2. Then peel the cucumber, cube it and place it over the top. Now blend the ingredients for around 1-2 minutes to incorporate them.

3. Finally pour the shake into a grass and serve.

Avocado Salsa

Prep Time: 10 minutes

Cook Time: 0 minutes

Total Time: 10 minutes

Calories 86.4, Carb 7.2g, Protein 1.3g, Fat 6.7g

Serves 4

Ingredients

1/8 cup cilantro

2 tablespoons fresh lime juice

1 California avocado

1 small red onion

1/2 jalapeno peppers

1 small whole red tomato

1/8 teaspoon each black pepper and salt

Directions

1. Chop the cilantro and tomato and set aside, then finely dice the jalapeno pepper and onion.

2. Then remove the skin from avocado, chop it and place into a serving bowl. Add in lime juice, jalapeno and the onion. Gently combine the avocado mixture.

3. Now fold the chopped cilantro and tomato and then season with salt and pepper.

4. Cover and chill until ready to be served.

Black Beauty – Low Carb Vodka Drink

Prep Time: 5 minutes

Cook Time: 0 minutes

Total time: 5 Minutes

Calories: 180, Carbs: 5g, Protein: 1g, Fat: 0g

Serves: 1 drink

Ingredients

Soda water

5 fresh mint leaves

¼ teaspoon ground black pepper

2 teaspoons powdered erythritol

¾ ounce fresh lemon juice (1 ½ tablespoons)

5 fresh blackberries

2 ounces vodka

Directions

1. Using ice, fill a large glass and set aside.

2. Then mix together mint leaves, black pepper, sweetener, lemon juice, black berries and vodka in a cocktail shaker.

3. Muddle the mixture until the mint and the fruit are crushed and have released respective juices.

4. At this point, strain the mixture of the cocktail shaker into the ice-filled glass.

5. Top the drink with soda water and garnish with fresh mint leaf and black berries.

Keto Dairy Free Shamrock

Prep Time: 5 minutes

Cook Time: 0 minutes

Total Time: 5 minutes

Calories: 259, Carbs: 7g, Protein: 26g, Fat: 14g

Serves 1

Ingredients

1 tablespoon of dark chocolate chips, sugar-free

5 drops of natural green food coloring

1/8 teaspoon peppermint extract

8 ice cubes

1/2 cup silk almond coconut milk

1 scoop vanilla protein powder, dairy free

1/2 medium avocado

Directions

1. Mix together ice, almond coconut milk, protein powder, avocado, food coloring and peppermint extract in a blender.

2. Pulse the contents until well incorporated and creamy, then top with sugar-free chocolate chips or dairy-free whipped cream if you like.

Asparagus and Leek Soup

Prep Time: 15 minutes

Cook Time: 15 minutes

Total Time: 30 minutes

Calories 167.7, Carbs 7.6g, Protein 4.9g, Fat 13.8g

Serves 1

Ingredients

1/3 cup heavy cream

1 14.5 oz. can chicken broth

1 teaspoons garlic

3/4 lb. asparagus

1 leek leek

2 tablespoons butter stick, unsalted

Directions

1. Into a large pot, melt butter over medium-high heat and then add in the leeks. Sauté for about 3 minutes and then add in the asparagus. Cook for a minute.

2. Then add in the garlic and sauté for additional 30 seconds.

3. Now add broth into the pot and let it boil. Reduce the heat and simmer for 8-10 minutes while covered.

4. Once the asparagus is tender, mix in the pepper and salt and then blend the soup in a processor to smoothness.

5. Return the soup to cooking pot to heat through before you serve. You can season with ground pepper and salt if required.

Low Carb Strawberry Margarita Gummy Worms

Prep Time: 10 minutes

Cook Time: 5 minutes

Total Time: 15 Minutes

Calories: 50, Carbs 2.6g, Protein 3.2g, Fat 0g

Serves 6

Ingredients

1 ½ ounces fresh lime juice

2 tablespoons powdered erythritol

3 tablespoons grass-fed gelatin collagen protein

2 ounces silver tequila

10 hulled strawberries, fresh or frozen

Directions

1. Mix together tequila and strawberries in a blender and process until smooth.

2. Then pour this mixture in medium pan and set over low heat. Add in lime juice, sweetener and gelatin and whisk until well dissolved.

4. Heat the mixture for 10 minutes as you whisk now and again until the mixture is fully pourable or thinner and smoother.

5. Move the mixture in a bowl that has a pour spout or a measuring cup

6. Instantly pour the mixture into a mold and put this in the fridge. Keep it chilled for about 10 minutes and then serve.

7. You should store any leftovers for up to week.

Salmon and Cream Cheese Bites

Prep Time 10 minutes

Cook Time 10 minutes

Total Time 20 minutes

Calories 32, Carbs 0.4g, Protein 1.9g, Fat 2.2g

Serves 4

Ingredients

50 grams cream cheese

1 teaspoon dried dill

50g fresh or smoked salmon slices

50g shredded/grated cheese

1/2 teaspoon salt

250 ml coconut milk or coconut cream

6 medium sized eggs

Directions

1. In a large pouring jug, whisk together eggs, coconut milk and salt and then fold in dill, smoked salmon, grated cheese and chopped cream cheese.

2. Pour the batter into greased silicon molds or mini muffin trays. Bake the mixture at about 180 degrees C for about 10 to 15 minutes.

3. Allow to cool and then serve.

Vanilla Pumpkin Seed Clusters

Prep Time: 5 minutes

Cook Time: 15 minutes

Total Time: 20 minutes

Calories 25, Carbs 1g, Protein 1g, Fat 2g

Serves: 30

Ingredients

Water, boiled

2 teaspoons coconut sugar

2 teaspoons honey

1 teaspoon vanilla extract

½ cup pumpkin seeds

Directions

1. Preheat an oven to 150 degrees Celsius, as you combine vanilla, coconut sugar and honey in a small bowl.

2. Stir together to produce thick paste, before adding a drop of boiled water; so as to create runny syrup. Pour the pumpkin seeds and stir to evenly coat the seeds.

3. Dollop a teaspoon of pumpkin seeds onto a baking sheet, and repeat the operation until it's all used up.

4. Cook the contents for about 15-20 minutes to brown the seeds. Remove from the oven and cool for some time.

5. After cooling, press the clusters together to ensure they don't fall apart. This will help them to dry quickly. Serve once cool and dry.

Pan-Fried Asparagus

Prep Time: 5 minutes

Cook Time: 15 minutes

Total Time: 20 minutes

Calories: 188, Carbs: 5.2g Protein: 2.8g, Fat: 18.4G

Serves 4

Ingredients

3 minced cloves of garlic

1/4 teaspoon of ground black pepper,

1 teaspoon of coarse salt

1/4 cup of butter

1 pound of fresh asparagus spears, trimmed

2 tablespoons of olive oil

Directions

1. In a skillet, melt some butter over medium-high heat.

2. Stir in olive oil, pepper and salt and cook garlic inside the butter for around 1 minute. Ensure that the garlic doesn't brown.

3. Now add in asparagus and continue to cook in the skillet for about 10 minutes. Ensure that you regularly turn asparagus to cook evenly.

Low Carb Egg Salad

Prep Time: minutes

Cook Time: minutes

Total Time: minutes

Calories 219, Protein 13.95 g, Fat 16.89 g, Carbs 1.91 g

Serves: 4

Ingredients

Pepper

Kosher salt

¼ teaspoon lite salt

1 teaspoon lemon juice

1 teaspoon Dijon mustard

2 tablespoon mayonnaise

6 eggs

Directions

1. First set the eggs in a saucepan, and then when done, add in cold water to cover to around 1 inch.

2. Boil the eggs for 10 minutes, and then remove from heat to cool. Under cold running water, peel the eggs and add them into a magic bullet or food processor. Blend until well chopped.

3. Then stir in the mayonnaise, pepper, salt and lemon juice and adjust the seasonings as desired.

4. If you like it, serve with bacon for wrapping and lettuce leaves.

Ketogenic Egg Cups

Prep time: 3 minutes

Cook time: 15 minutes

Total time: 18 minutes

Calories 174, Carbs 1.12g, Protein 11.86g, Fat 13.14g

Serves: 12

Ingredients

8 asparagus spears, chopped

12 strips uncured organic bacon, cooked

12 eggs

Coconut oil or ghee

Black pepper

Sea Salt

Directions

1. Heat the oven to 400 degrees F. Meanwhile, grease about 12 cups of a muffin pan.

2. Then lay a bacon strip in each cup, and push it down so that it doesn't hang outside.

3. Crack an egg in each muffin cup and distribute the asparagus in each. Add some salt and pepper then bake in the middle of the oven for about 15 minutes.

4. Serve the eggs warm or keep cooled until ready to serve.

Thyme-lemon Garlic Mushrooms

Prep Time: 5 minutes

Cook Time: 10 minutes

Total Time: 15 minutes

Calories 73, Carbs 2g, Protein 0.1g, Fat 7.5g

Serves: 2-3

Ingredients

1 tablespoon coconut oil or olive oil

1 teaspoon ghee

Zest of 1 lemon + a drizzle of lemon juice

1 garlic clove, peeled and diced

5 springs of fresh thyme, leaves only

10-11oz sliced button mushrooms

Black pepper and sea salt

Directions

1. In a large frying pan, heat some coconut oil until hot and then add in thyme and mushrooms.

2. Cook the mixture on high until browned of for about 3 to 4 minutes. As soon as they begin to shrink slightly and produce a fluid, flip the ingredients and cook for another 2 minutes or so.

3. At this point, add in garlic, pepper, lemon zest, thyme, butter and sea salt and cook for about 1 or 2 minutes while stirring occasionally.

4. Now add in more fresh thyme and a drizzle of fresh lemon juice if you like it.

Desserts

Mock Cinnabon

Prep Time: 5 minutes

Cook Time: 0 minutes

Total Time: 5 minutes

Calories

Serves 4

Ingredients

7 pecans halves, toasted

1 packets splenda

1/2 cups cottage cheese

1 drop maple extract or other sugar-substitute

Ground cinnamon

Directions

1. Combine maple extract, cottage cheese and the sugar substitute then sprinkle with cinnamon.

2. Top the dessert with pecan halves.

Baked Cream Cheese

Prep Time: 10 minutes

Cook Time: 15 minutes

Total Time: 25 minutes

Calories 159, Carbs 6.4g, Protein 3.4g, Fat 13.3g

Serves 8

Ingredients

1/2 teaspoon dried dill weed

1 egg yolk, beaten

1/2 (8-ounce) package refrigerated crescent roll (keto friendly)

1 (8-ounce) package cream cheese

Directions

1. Preheat your oven to 350°F.

2. On a lightly floured surface, unroll the dough and then press together the seams to form 12x4 inch rectangle.

3. Use half of the dill to sprinkle one side of the cream cheese. In the center of the dough, put a brick of cream cheese with the dill side down and then proceed to sprinkle some dill on top of cream cheese.

4. Now bring the sides of the dough together to enclose the cream cheese and then press the edges to seal it.

5. Put the dough onto a lightly greased cookie sheet and then brush using a beaten egg.

6. At this point, bake the cream cheese into preheated oven for about 15-18 minutes. Serve it while warm.

Fried Honey Banana

Prep Time: 5 minutes

Cook Time: 5 minutes

Total Time: 10 minutes

Calories 146, Carbs 12g, Protein 0.73g, Fat 7.01g

Serves 2

Ingredients

Serves 1

1 tablespoon olive oil or coconut oil

1 teaspoon cinnamon

1 tablespoon organic honey

1 banana, sliced

1 tablespoon water

Directions

1. In a skillet, lightly heat coconut oil over medium heat.

2. Then arrange your banana slices in the skillet and cook for around 1-2 minutes on each side.

3. As the banana slices cook, whisk a tablespoon of water and organic honey.

4. Take out the pan from heat and now pour in your honey mixture over the sliced cooked bananas.

4. Once cool, sprinkle with cinnamon and serve.

Black Olives with Cheddar

Prep Time: 5 minutes

Cook Time: 0 minutes

Total Time: 5 minutes

Calories 223, Carbs 6.8g, Protein 7.9g, Fat 19.3g

Serves 1

Ingredients

1 slice cheddar cheese

7 Greek olives black olives

Directions

1. Dice the cheese and put into the hole in the olive.

2. Pop them into the mouth and enjoy.

White Chocolate Fat Bomb

Prep Time 5 minutes

Cook Time 10 minutes

Total Time 15 minutes

Calories 125, Carbs 0g, Protein 0g, Fat 10g

Serves 8

Ingredients

10 drops vanilla stevia drops

1/4 cup coconut oil (about 35g)

1/4 cup cocoa butter (about 25g)

Directions

1. Melt together coconut oil and cocoa butter in a double boiler or in a skillet over low heat.

2. Then remove from heat and stir in a few stevia drops. Pour the mixture into molds and keep it refrigerated until hardened or ready to serve.

3. To serve, remove from the molds and store any remainder in the fridge.

Baby Greens with Grapefruit and Red Onion

Prep Time: 15 minutes

Cook Time: 0 minutes

Total Time: 15 minutes

Calories 146.1, Carbs 13.5g, Protein 1.7g, Fat 10.3g

Serves 4

Ingredients

1/2 small red onions

3.75 cups spring mix salad

1 teaspoon leaves tarragon

3 tablespoons extra virgin olive oil

1/4 teaspoon yellow mustard seed

1 fruit grapefruit (pink and red)

Directions

1. Begin by cutting the grape fruit into sections. Then set aside the sections while reserving about 1 tablespoon of grapefruit juice.

2. To a mixing bowl, add in the grapefruit juice along with mustard. Drizzle in some oil and whisk well to blend.

3. Then stir in tarragon, salt and black pepper, and now set aside.

4. At this point, add in the greens and toss with the salad dressing, red onion and the grapefruit sections.

146.1 Calories, 1.7g Protein, 10.3g Fat, 13.5g carbs

Instant Pot Chocolate Fondue

Prep Time: 2 minutes

Cook Time: 10 minutes

Total Time: 12 minutes

Calories: 216, Carbs: 11.7g, Protein: 1.8g, Fat: 20.3g

Serves 2-4

Ingredients

1 teaspoon Amaretto liquor

1 teaspoon coconut sugar

3.5 oz. fresh cream

3.5 oz. Swiss dark bittersweet chocolate 85%

Directions

1. Add 2 cups of water and a rack to Instant Pot and set aside.

2. Add the chocolate in large chunks in a heat-prove container and obtain their weight.

3. Add same amount of sugar, fresh cream, liquor and spices if desired.

4. Lower the container into Instant Pot and lock the lid. Cook for 2 minutes on high pressure then quick release pressure.

5. Pull out the container using tongs then stir the contents for a minute using a fork. Do this to create a thick dark-brown mixture.

6. Serve with fresh fruit preferably sliced into bite-sizes.

Chocolate Almond Keto Fat Bomb

Prep Time: 5 minutes

Cook Time: 0 minutes

Total Time: 5 minutes

Calories: 260, Carbs: 6g, Protein: 4g, Fat: 26g

Serves: 15

Ingredients

10-15 whole almonds

½ cup cacao powder

1 cup coconut oil

1/4 cup coconut flour

1 cup almond butter

Directions

1. In a saucepan, melt some coconut oil and butter. Add in stevia, coconut flour and cacao powder and mix well.

2. Allow the mixture to cool down and then make 10 to 15 ping-pong sized balls from the batter.

3. Now stick an almond into each bomb and keep it refrigerated until ready to serve.

Coconut Avocado Mousse

Prep Time: 10 minutes

Cook Time: 0 minutes

Total Time: 10 minutes

Calories: 204, Carbs: 21g, Protein: 3g, Fat: 14g

Serves 1

Ingredients

Cacao nibs for topping

1/2 cup young coconut flesh

1/2 ripe avocado

Directions

1. Add all the three ingredients into a high speed blender.

2. Add in a dash of coconut water or filtered water if you like it.

3. Now pour the mixture into a glass and serve. Garnish with chocolate chunks or cacao nibs if you like.

Nut Free Keto Brownie

Prep Time 10 minutes

Cook Time 20 minutes

Total Time 30 minutes

Calories 178, Carbs 3.5g, Protein 4.5g, Fat 17g

Servings 12

Ingredients

4.2 ounces cream cheese, softened

3 - 5 tablespoons granulated sweetener

2 teaspoons vanilla

1/2 teaspoon baking powder

2.2 ounces cocoa, unsweetened

5.6 ounces butter, melted

6 eggs

Directions

1. In a mixing bowl, put all the ingredients and blend into smoothness using a stick blender with blade attachment.

2. Pour the batter into a 21 by 8.5 inch baking dish. Bake at 350 degrees F until well cooked at the center. This should take around 20-15 minutes.

3. Slice the brownie into squares, triangle wedges or rectangle bars and serve.

Secret Ingredient Chocolate Mousse

Prep Time: 15 minutes

Cook Time: 0 minutes

Total Time: 15 minutes

Calories 192, Carbs: 4.2g, Protein: 2.4g, Fat: 17.7g

Serves: 8

Ingredients

2-3 tablespoons Swerve sweetener

⅛ teaspoon vanilla extract

8 ounces cream cheese block, softened

½ large avocado, pitted

Optional garnish 90% dark chocolate shaved,

¼ cup cocoa powder, unsweetened

¼ cup heavy whipping cream

Directions

1. Using a handheld mixer, beat cream cheese in a medium mixing bowl until smooth and creamy.

2. Mix in cocoa powder and beat in avocado. Continue to mix until fully incorporated, or for around 5 minutes.

3. Add in the sweetener and vanilla extract and beat for 1-2 minutes, or until smooth.

4. Whip heavy cream into a bowl until stiff peaks form. Put the whipped cream inside the prepared chocolate mixture and then proceed to gently fold to blend.

5. Next, place the chocolate mousse inside a piping bag then proceed to pipe it into the different containers. You can use the dark chocolate shavings to garnish if you like.

Berries with Chocolate Ganache

Prep Time: 10 minutes

Cook Time: 5 minutes

Total Time: 15 minutes

Calories 286.3, Carbs 8.1g, Protein 4g, Fat 17.6g

Serves 6

Ingredients

8 oz. strawberries

2 cups red raspberries

2 cups fresh blueberries

8 ounce chocolate chips, sugar free

1/3 cup heavy cream

1/2 teaspoons vanilla extract

Directions

1. Mix together the fruits and put into dessert bowls.

2. Heat the heavy cream and chocolate chips over low heat until melted, or microwave the mixture for around 30 seconds.

3. Then add the vanilla and stir to get a smooth consistency.

4. Cool slightly and then serve.

Conclusion

We have come to the end of the book. Thank you for reading and congratulations for reading until the end.

I truly hope this book has opened your eyes to the possibility that you can follow the Ketogenic diet irrespective of how busy you are, as you can prepare something for breakfast, lunch, dinner, snack or even a dessert within as little as 30 minutes using not more than 7 ingredients! What you need to do next is to take action; experiment with the many recipes in this book to find what you like most then after that, you can come up with your own meal plan.

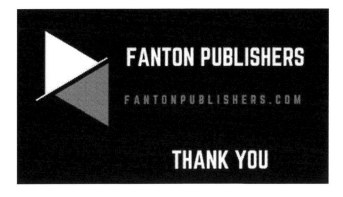

Do You Like My Book & Approach To Publishing?

If you like my writing and style and would love the ease of learning literally everything you can get your hands on from Fantonpublishers.com, I'd really need you to do me either of the following favors.

1: First, I'd Love It If You Leave a Review of This Book on Amazon.

2: Check Out My Other Keto Diet Books

KETOGENIC DIET: Keto Diet Made Easy: Beginners Guide on How to Burn Fat Fast With the Keto Diet (Including 100+ Recipes That You Can Prepare Within 20 Minutes)- New Edition

KETOGENIC DIET: Ketogenic Diet Recipes That You Can Prepare Using 7 Ingredients and Less in Less Than 30 Minutes

Ketogenic Diet: With A Sustainable Twist: Lose Weight Rapidly With Ketogenic Diet Recipes You Can Make Within 25 Minutes

Ketogenic Diet: Keto Diet Breakfast Recipes

Fat Bombs: Keto Fat Bombs: 50+ Savory and Sweet Ketogenic Diet Fat Bombs That You MUST Prepare Before Any Other!

Snacks: Keto Diet Snacks: 50+ Savory and Sweet Ketogenic Diet Snacks That You MUST Prepare Before Any Other!

Desserts: Keto Diet Desserts: 50+ Savory and Sweet Ketogenic Diet Desserts That You MUST Prepare Before Any Other!

Ketogenic Diet: Ketogenic Diet Lunch and Dinner Recipes

Ketogenic Diet: Keto Diet Cookbook For Vegetarians

Ketogenic Diet: Ketogenic Slow Cooker Cookbook: Keto Slow Cooker Recipes That You Can Prepare Using 7 Ingredients Or Less

Note: This list may not represent all my Keto diet books. You can check the full list by visiting my Author Central: amazon.com/author/fantonpublishers or my website http://www.fantonpublishers.com

Get updates when we publish any book on the Ketogenic diet: http://bit.ly/2fantonpubketo

Closely related to the keto diet is intermittent fasting. I also publish books on Intermittent Fasting.

One of the books is shown below:

Intermittent Fasting: A Complete Beginners Guide to Intermittent Fasting For Weight Loss, Increased Energy, and A Healthy Life

Get updates when we publish any book on intermittent fasting: http://bit.ly/2fantonbooksIF

To get a list of all my other books, please fantonwriters.com, my author central or let me send you the list by requesting them below: http://bit.ly/2fantonpubnewbooks

3: Let's Get In Touch

Antony

Website: http://www.fantonpublishers.com/

Email: Support@fantonpublishers.com

Twitter: https://twitter.com/FantonPublisher

Facebook Page: https://www.facebook.com/Fantonpublisher/

My Ketogenic Diet Books Page: https://www.facebook.com/pg/Fast-Keto-Meals-336338180266944

Private Facebook Group For Readers: https://www.facebook.com/groups/FantonPublishers/

Pinterest: https://www.pinterest.com/fantonpublisher/

4: Grab Some Freebies On Your Way Out; Giving Is Receiving, Right?

I gave you 2 freebies at the start of the book, one on general life transformation and one about the Ketogenic diet. Grab them here if you didn't grab them earlier.

Ketogenic Diet Freebie: http://bit.ly/2fantonpubketo

5 Pillar Life Transformation Checklist: http://bit.ly/2fantonfreebie

5: Suggest Topics That You'd Love Me To Cover To Increase Your Knowledge Bank. I am looking forward to seeing your suggestions and insights; you could even suggest improvements to this book. Simply send me a message on Support@fantonpublishers.com.

PSS: Let Me Also Help You Save Some Money!

If you are a heavy reader, have you considered subscribing to Kindle Unlimited? You can read this and millions of other books for just $9.99 a month)! You can check it out by searching for Kindle Unlimited on Amazon!

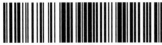

Printed in Great Britain
by Amazon